Everything You Need to Know About

CREATING YOUR OWN SUPPORT SYSTEM

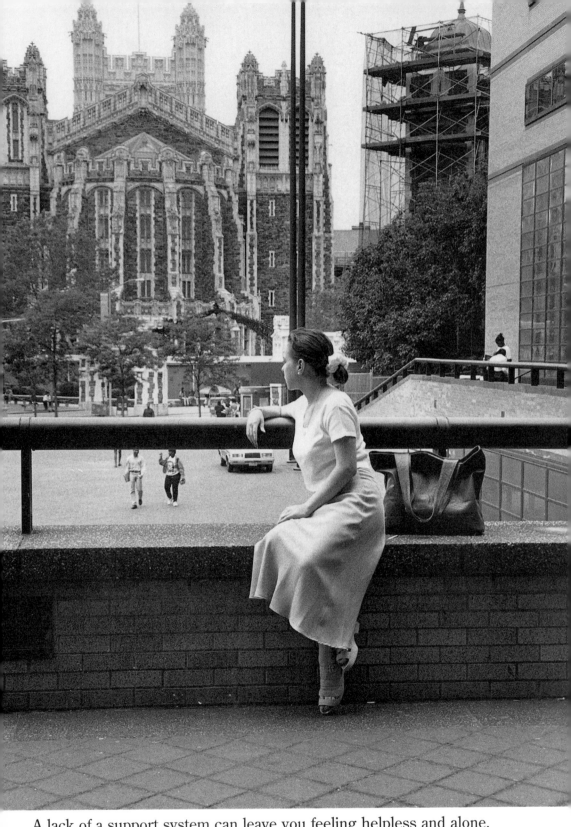

A lack of a support system can leave you feeling helpless and alone.

Everything You Need to Know About

CREATING YOUR OWN SUPPORT SYSTEM

Anna Kreiner

THE ROSEN PUBLISHING GROUP, INC.
NEW YORK

Published in 1996 by The Rosen Publishing Group, Inc.
29 East 21st Street, New York, NY 10010

First Edition

Manufactured in the United States of America

Library of Congress Cataloging-in-Publication Data

Kreiner, Anna.
    Everything you need to know about creating your own support system /
Anna Kreiner. — 1st ed.
      p. cm. — (The need to know library)
    Includes bibliographical references and index.
    Summary: Discusses how teenagers can create their own support
system, a group of people in their lives to whom they feel connected
and who can help them build skills and solve problems.
    ISBN 0-8239-2215-4
    1. Teenagers—Social networks—United States—Juvenile literature.
[1. Social networks. 2. Interpersonal relations.] I. Title.
II. Series.
HQ796.K693   1996
646.7'00835—dc20
                                                  95-10753
                                                     CIP
                                                        AC

Contents

Introduction

*C*harlie reached out his hand and banged on the alarm clock. Why should he even bother to get out of bed? School would be boring. The teachers didn't care about him. Sometimes he played basketball with a few of the guys after school, but he didn't have any real friends. Mostly he just hung out on his own, bored and lonely.

Lately things hadn't been too great at home either. Ever since Dad left six months ago, Mom had been busy working and taking care of his younger sister, Lois. At night she either ignored him or yelled at him. He wasn't sure which was worse.

Charlie threw off the covers and dragged himself out of bed. He guessed he would go to school. But he didn't think anyone would care if he stayed in bed all day. Or maybe all year.

Have you ever felt the way Charlie did that morning? He thinks no one cares about him or his future. Charlie doesn't have a support system.

Your support system is the group of people in your life to whom you feel connected. They help you by giving you guidance, education, and support. It's important to have a strong support system so that you can grow, cope with your problems, and reach your goals.

Who provides this help? Many different kinds of people may be in your support system. Parents, brothers and sisters, cousins, aunts, uncles, and other relatives often play a big role in your network.

But even if you had no family, you could have a support system. Classmates, teachers and guidance counselors, youth leaders, and neighbors are some of the other people who can help you too.

Having a support system is important because we all need other people. Sometimes they teach you new skills—in the classroom, on the job, or in the community. Friends encourage you when you face challenges, and they listen when you have a problem. Older relatives or other adults can use their experience to offer advice or serve as role models. They may help you find a job or plan for the future.

Creating a good support system is one of the most important things you can do for yourself. Then you will be able to look to other people for help and guidance. The particular persons in your network may change, but you will always be interacting with others. Once you know how to build a strong support system, you will be able to use these skills for the rest of your life.

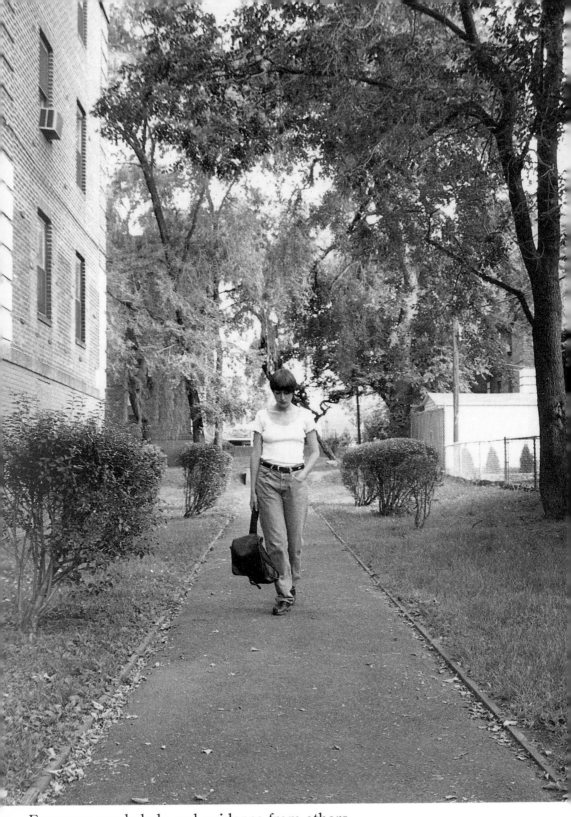

Everyone needs help and guidance from others.

Chapter 1

What Is a Support System?

A support system is a network of individuals or groups in your life who help you work toward your goals. These people assist you in setting goals, increasing your confidence, and learning new skills.

We couldn't live without other people. They help us get the basic necessities—food, clothing, and shelter. But we also need encouragement, sympathy, and guidance. That's what a good support system provides for you.

The people in your network offer emotional support—in good times and bad. They can also help you find a job, continue your education, and develop your talents.

Unfortunately, many teens do not have a strong support system. Without a network of people around you, you will not be able to meet all your needs. You may feel without direction, lonely, and frustrated.

But you can build a strong social support system for yourself. This book will help you develop the skills you need to build your own support network.

The people in your support system can teach you many things. Sometimes you may learn specific skills. Your English teacher will help you improve your writing ability. You can learn how to throw a fastball from your baseball coach.

Sometimes the people in your support system will work with you to reach your goals. If you want to earn money, your neighbor may help you create a strategy to find and get a job. Are you thinking about what you want to do after you finish high school? Talk to your cousin who recently graduated and plans to start college in the fall.

Older people can use their experiences to tell you about choices they have made and the effects these decisions have had on their lives. You may use their advice when you make your own choices.

Judy wasn't sure what to do. She wanted to earn extra money to save for college. But she was afraid that if she spent too many hours working she wouldn't have enough time to study.

Finally she decided to ask her neighbor, Mrs. Alvarez, for advice. Mrs. Alvarez told Maria that when she was in high school she had worked in the library. The job helped her save for college and

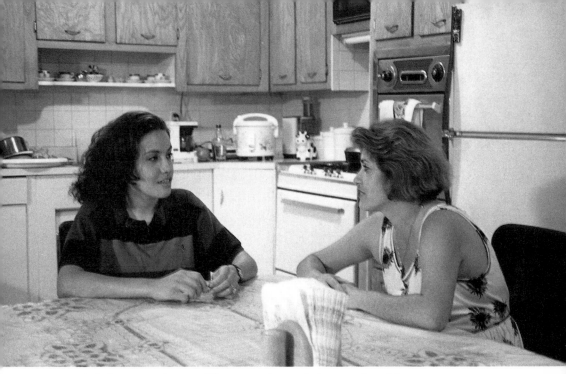

Adults are often willing to give advice and guidance to teenagers.

allowed her time to study. And she had plenty of books to read!

Mrs. Alvarez helped Judy apply for a position at the local library. Today Judy works there several hours a week, saves money for college, and still has time to keep up her studies.

In this case Judy's support system helped her because she relied on the advice of a role model. She applied Mrs. Alvarez's experience to her own situation. Then she formed a plan to reach her goals.

The people in your support system can assist you in deciding what is important to you and planning for the future. Talking to other people

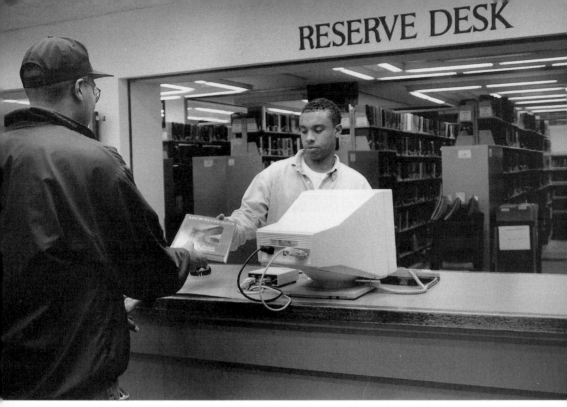

An activity, such as a part-time job, is one way to interact with new people.

may help you to decide on your goals. They can also work with you to identify your strengths and weaknesses.

Becoming involved with other people can help you build your self-esteem. They may praise you for your talents, your good behavior, or your accomplishments. After you've succeeded with one project, you'll know you can use those skills in the future. You'll also feel good about yourself when you know you're helping others.

Marla used to walk home from school and hide in her room. She had a slight stutter and was embarrassed to talk to other people. She was afraid they would laugh at her or not understand what she was saying.

One afternoon her neighbor, Mrs. Jeffers, asked Marla if she would help her give a party for her three-year-old son. At first Marla was afraid of being teased. But she loves children so she agreed to do the work.

Soon Marla got so involved with the preparations that she forgot to be self-conscious.

"Marla," said Mrs. Jeffers after the party was over. "You did a wonderful job. I'm going to recommend you to my friends."

Soon Marla was helping other people with their parties. They loved her work, and Marla recognized that she had a special talent. She was less embarrassed to be with other people. She started to spend more time with her classmates.

She still has a stutter, but other people can understand what she says. And most important, she doesn't let it bother her.

Her increased self-confidence has helped her to establish connections with more people. From that first step, her support network is getting bigger and stronger.

You'll often find that once you start to build your own support system it almost seems to grow by itself. You develop connections with a few people, and soon you're interacting with more and more. The greater the number of people with whom you

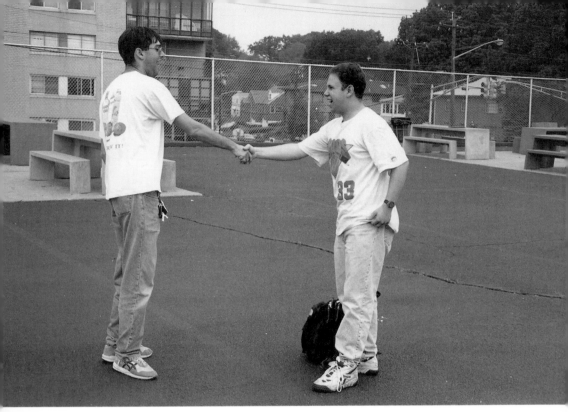

One of the advantages of a support system is that you can
provide support to others who have helped you.

can connect, the more likely you are to get the
support and connections you need.

A Two-Way Street

You gain many advantages from a support
system, but it is a two-way street. At the same time
that you get assistance from other people, you also
help them.

The people in your network give and take.
During the spring you volunteered to help Mr.
O'Connor in his garden shop. He thought you
were very reliable, and he liked your work.

Suppose you want to apply for a full-time position at the local nursery after you graduate. Because you did a good job in his store, Mr. O'Connor will probably agree to write a letter of recommendation for you.

Getting a part-time job or volunteering in your community can help you build your support system. You will gain skills and self-confidence and learn about different kinds of work. You can add these new abilities to your list of qualifications when you write a résumé or fill out a job application.

Your employers or supervisors will become an important part of your support network, especially when you are ready for a full-time job. They will probably be glad to act as references or tell potential employers about your talents. They can offer suggestions about finding the job you want, and they may be able to introduce you to other businesspeople who are looking for workers.

After Rebecca's grandfather died, she felt very lonely. She decided to volunteer in a nursing home. Every week Rebecca visited Mr. Jones. The two of them became part of each other's support network. Mr. Jones depended on Rebecca to help him with his daily living skills. He also liked to hear about her activities.

At the same time, Rebecca gained from her relationship with Mr. Jones. Her self-esteem

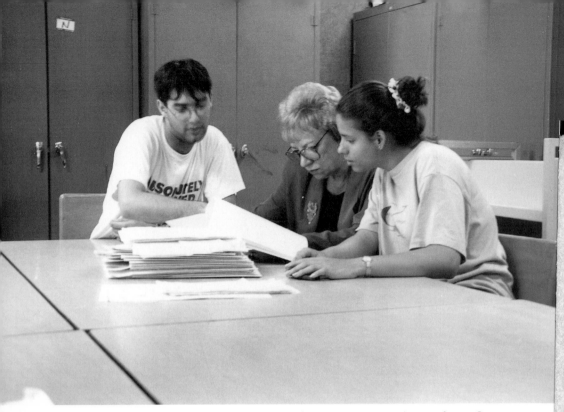

Working with older people can be an opportunity to benefit from their life experience.

increased because she knew she was doing a good job. Mr. Jones offered her good advice when she had a problem. Both Rebecca and Mr. Jones gained from their interactions.

Rebecca also got to know the staff at the nursing home. She especially liked the physical therapist and began to volunteer as an aide in his department. She decided that after graduating from high school she wanted to become a physical therapist. Because Rebecca was such a reliable and productive worker, her supervisor offered to write a supportive letter when Rebecca applied to physical therapy school.

You know that a good support system provides companionship, guidance, and education. You can also use your support system to find a job, learn new skills, and make vocational and educational plans. Now it's time to learn who can be a part of that network.

Who Is in Your Support Network?

Your support system may include many kinds of people. Friends, relatives, neighbors, clergypeople, teachers, counselors, and local businesspeople are some of the most important people who could be in your network. Some of these people you know already. With others you may have to use more effort, by joining an organization, volunteering, getting a job, writing a letter, or simply introducing yourself to them.

Each person in your support system has a special role to play. Not everyone will meet all of your needs. And some people will help you in more ways than one. For example, you might learn how to dribble from your basketball coach and how to repair furniture from your shop teacher. If you respect and admire your coach, you might also be able to talk to him when you're having problems at home. The owner of the local supermarket may be able to offer you a part-time job that will give you extra pocket money and teach you valuable skills to use in the future.

Because you have many needs, it's important to include different kinds of people in your support system. You don't need crowds of people in your life to have a strong network. Usually, the more people with whom you feel connected, the more likely you are to meet your needs.

Chapter 2
Why Do I Feel Alone?

It's hard to be alone. Other people in your life can provide emotional support, education, and increased self-esteem. A good support system is very important.

But many teens don't have a strong network of people around them. Some young people spend most of their time by themselves. And even teens who seem to have friends may not feel connected to anyone. These young people live very much alone.

Many teens need direction in their lives. What kind of job do you want to have when you finish high school? Will you need more education? Who can help you make these important decisions?

Your support system can help you plan for the future. Many businesspeople are well-established members of your community. You will benefit from their knowledge and experience. They can offer

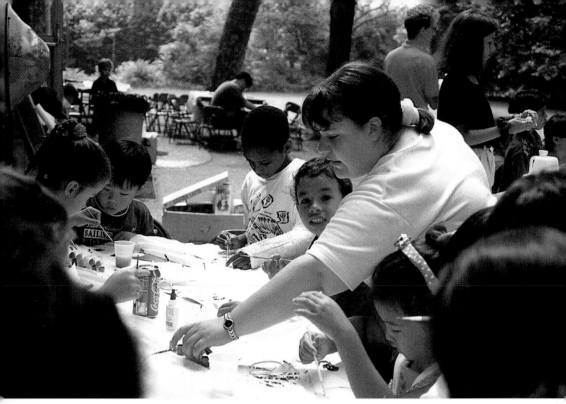

Sometimes, children can grow up without a strong support system even as they are surrounded by people.

advice and introduce you to people who do the kind of work you like. They may be willing to write letters of recommendation or help you fill out college or job applications.

Just being with other people doesn't guarantee that you will have a strong support network. It's possible to be surrounded by others and still not feel that your needs are being met. You might hang out with your pals after school and eat dinner with your family every night, but do you have a support system?

If you don't think you can talk to anyone about your problems or get help and encouragement when you want it, you are not getting the emotional support you need.

It's important to make connections to fill your other needs too. You can't get advice from a counselor if you don't go to the career guidance office. Your employer won't know you want a letter of recommendation unless you ask her. You have to tell the people around you what you want so that they can help you.

Problems at Home

There are many reasons that you may not have a strong support system in place.

Sometimes teens live in troubled families and can't get the support they need from their parents or brothers and sisters. If your mom drinks too much or your father is abusive, they probably will not be available to help you. Your brothers and sisters may be preoccupied with their own problems.

Sometimes it seems that at the very times you most need help there's no one to support you. But that isn't true. There are many other people who can give you help when you need it.

If your relatives can't be part of your support system, it's important for you to look to people outside your family. Later in this book you'll learn how you can find others to become part of your social support system.

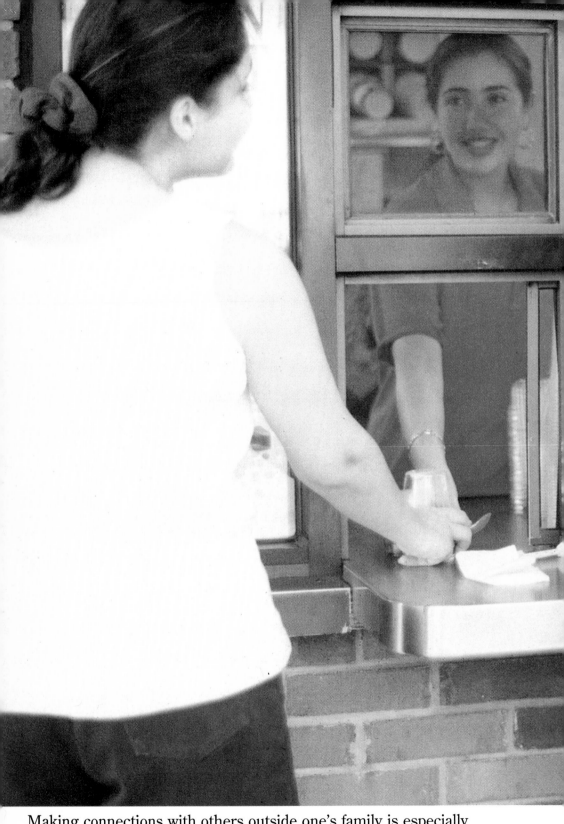

Making connections with others outside one's family is especially important for teens who have problems at home.

Knowing Your Needs

Some teens don't have a strong support system because they haven't identified their needs. In order to develop a good support system for yourself you have to know what you want and how other people can help you.

Identifying your needs is a key step in creating a good support system. But just as important is finding people who can help you in meeting those needs. Some teens have no support network because they don't know where to get help.

For example, you may have a goal to continue your education after you finish high school, but you don't know whom you should ask for help.

Guidance counselors, youth leaders, and teachers are good resource people. They can help you identify your goals and develop a strategy for carrying out your plan. Besides giving you information, they may also put you in touch with other people who could become part of your support system.

You may be bothered by a family problem and want to talk to someone, but you're embarrassed and don't know whom to ask. Try talking to a cousin or an aunt. Perhaps a classmate or a teacher you trust will listen to your problems.

If you want to get a job, talk to people in the community who do the kind of work you like. They may have a position or know someone else who can help you.

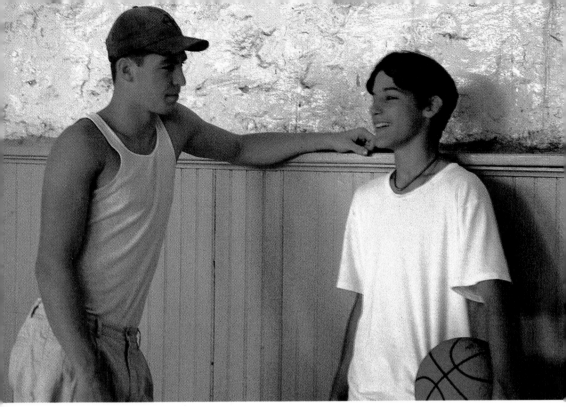

People are often happy to help you if you approach them
honestly and directly.

Once you know what you want from other
people, think about the people you know who
might be able to help you. Trust your instincts,
and don't be afraid to ask for help. Even if the
person you first approach can't help you, he or she
may be able to refer you to someone else who can.

Your support system can be the key to a
successful future. Teachers, mentors, and
employers can help you gain experience and
develop your abilities. You'll gain confidence and
acquire skills to use in the future. Through your
network you'll have the opportunity to meet other

people who share your interests. They may be able to guide you in getting the education and experience you need to start yourself in a satisfying career.

Creating a strong support system takes work. But the effort you make will provide many benefits. Developing these skills will give you rewards to last a lifetime.

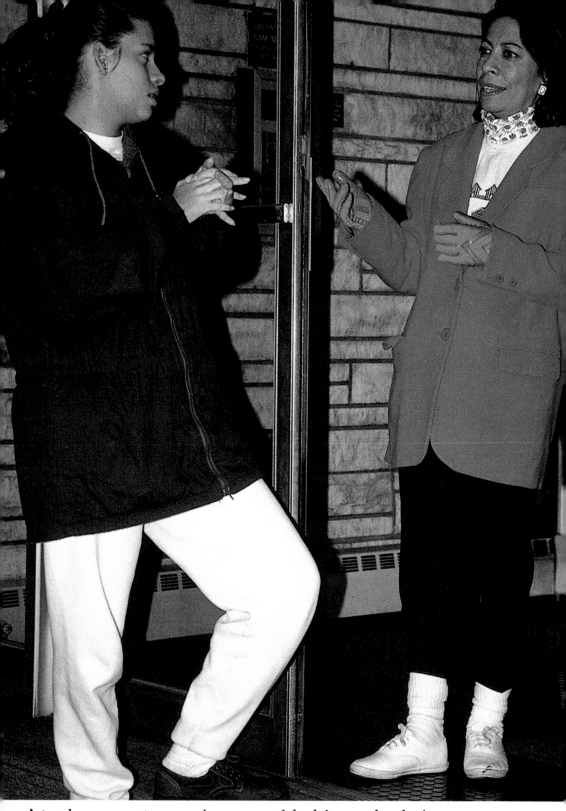

A teacher or mentor can give you useful advice on developing your skills and abilities.

Chapter 3

Creating Your Support Network

Before you develop your support network, it's important to figure out what you want to get from it. You have to identify your needs.

You might start by making a list of the most important things you hope to get from the people around you. Will working with others increase your confidence? Do you want help in planning your education? Will your employer serve as a reference for you? Can a local entrepreneur tell you about how she started her own business? Your list might include: increased self-esteem, emotional support, new skills, companionship, career guidance. You can add other items to your list. Think about what you don't have that other people can help you attain.

Do You Have a Support System Now?

Once you know what you want, decide whether or not you are getting these things from the people around you. Are the people in your life working as a support system for you?

One of the best ways to get what you want is to ask for it directly. You may not be getting support from others because they don't know what you need. You are most likely to succeed if you tell them specifically what you want and how they can help you.

Heidi loved sports, and she loved listening to the radio. She thought she might like to be a sports reporter after she finished high school. But she didn't know how to get started. So she wrote a letter to the baseball commentator on her favorite radio station and asked for his advice. He offered to give her a tour of the station and explained how he began his career as a reporter.

Heidi benefited by taking the time to communicate clearly. In her letter she told the broadcaster what she wanted, and he was able to help her. Many people are willing to give you their time and energy if they understand what you want.

You can build your communication skills through practice. Try writing letters or speaking in front of small groups. You might join the debate

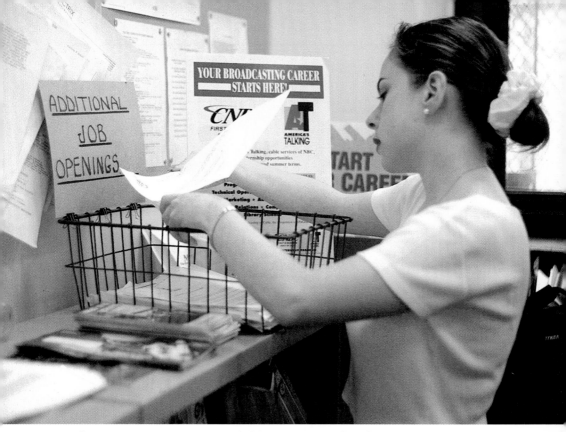

There are resources available at your school or community center to help you get organized and plan for the future.

team or the drama club. Volunteering to teach younger children or working in a hospital will also help you to communicate well with others.

Using Your Resources Wisely

Your guidance counselor can help you make plans for life after high school. Ask your math teacher where you can get extra tutoring if you need it. The youth leader at your community center will be glad to tell you about the recreation classes starting in the fall.

It's important to know who can help you and

whether you are interacting with them in the best possible way to create a strong support system for yourself.

Harold was thinking about the kind of work he would do after high school. He wasn't sure what his skills were or where to start planning for a career. And he didn't know who could help him. Finally he told his friend Joe about his problems.

"Job help?" said Joe. "Don't you know about the vocational center in the guidance office? You can talk to the counselors there. They'll give you an aptitude test to help you figure out jobs that would fit you. And they offer advice on getting the job you want."

Harold had never known about the career office. He made an appointment to meet with one of the counselors. The advisor helped Harold identify several areas of interest and gave him information about how he could pursue these careers.

The counselor had been in his office the whole school year, but he didn't become part of Harold's support system until Harold made the appointment.

Harold learned an important lesson that afternoon. A key part of having a support system is using the resources available to you to meet your needs.

Chapter 4

Filling in the Gaps

Y ou've made a list of your needs and examined whether or not the people in your life are providing you with the right amount and kinds of support. The next step in creating your support network is to fill in the gaps. Identify those areas where you need more support and then think about who can help you.

Sometimes people who help you in one situation can provide other kinds of support too.

Family members and friends are often the easiest place to start building your support network. Try talking to your parents, brothers and sisters, aunts, uncles, or cousins. You know these people, and you may find it easier to talk to them than to strangers.

Your next-door neighbor always offers good advice when you and your mom have an argument. He is also a successful painter. Now you

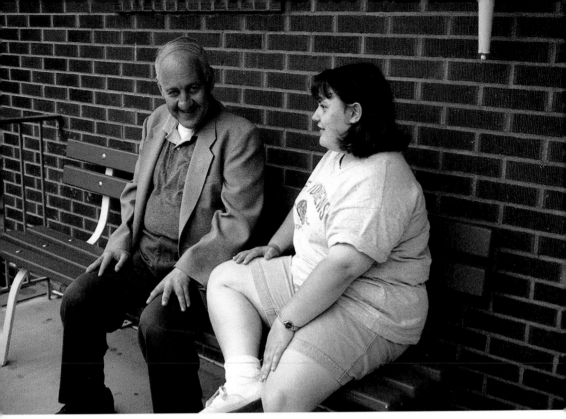

An individual who has experience in a field you are interested in can provide valuable guidance.

might talk to him about your plans to apply to art school after you finish high school.

Sometimes you can strengthen the ties with people who are already in your life. To meet other needs you may need to add people to your support network.

Suppose you want to feel better about yourself by assisting other people. It might be time for you to join a service club or become part of a volunteer program at the local hospital.

Han Lee was worried. It was almost the end of his junior year, and he didn't know what he would do after he finished high school.

One day Han Lee saw a flyer at the local YMCA advertising for an assistant at an after-school program for elementary school students. He likes helping people, and the younger kids at school often ask him for advice. So he decided to volunteer for the position.

Soon Han Lee's support system was growing fast! The younger students looked up to him. The youth leaders in the program praised him for his creativity and good planning skills. In May his supervisor offered him a paid position as a counselor for the summer camp at the YMCA.

By building his support network, Han Lee helped himself in many ways. He developed his leadership abilities, which he can use in the future. His volunteer position led to paid work. And he will probably be able to ask his supervisor for a letter of recommendation when he applies for another job or wants to continue his education. He also gained useful contacts through the parents of the children he taught. One parent, for example, was a museum curator and offered Han a part-time job leading groups of students around the museum on weekends.

You can work on your leadership skills by becoming part of the Scouts or a youth group at your community center. You might also join a career-oriented club like the Junior Achievement League or Future Teachers of America. Ask your

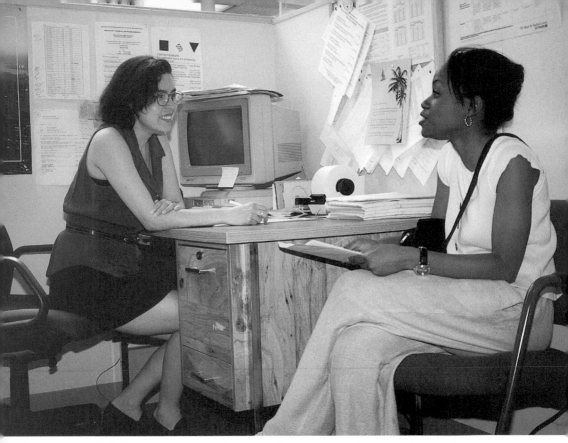

Talking to a counselor or advisor can give you ideas for planning your future.

guidance counselor or youth center leader for information about these groups or others like them. Look in the library for a list of local organizations.

Looking Outside Your Family

Families are a good place for many teens to get support, but sometimes relatives can't or won't help you.

You don't have to rely on your family to have a support system. Set up an appointment to meet with a guidance counselor or one of your favorite teachers at school. Talk to a youth leader, a neighbor, or a local businessperson. Often these people can help you with your problems. They may also be able to suggest other individuals or groups who can become part of your network.

If your family belongs to a religious organization, you might contact the priest, minister, rabbi, or youth leader of your congregation. Check the local youth center or community club in your neighborhood for teen groups and older mentors.

"I wanted to have a good life after high school. But I was scared. I didn't know if I could handle getting a job, living on my own, and taking care of myself. And there's no one at home who has the time to help me figure out what to do," said Lila.

One afternoon she noticed a sign on the bulletin board at the grocery store. The local Boys and Girls Club was offering a "Life After High School" program. The counselors there would help teens like Lila prepare for independent living.

"The counselors were great. We had classes on how to find a job and set up our own apartment. We each had our own advisor. The counselors led groups for teens to talk about what scares us. They helped us make plans for the future and deal with our problems.

"The people in the program became like a second

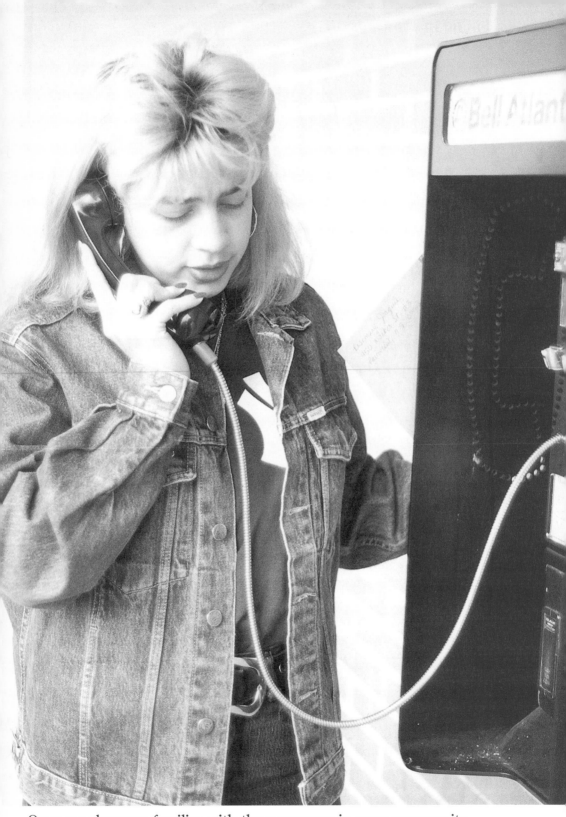

Once you become familiar with the resources in your community,
you will know whom to call with questions or problems.

*family to me," said Lila. "They helped me make
plans, and they kept track of my progress. And I
know I can always turn to them for support if I need
it in the future."*

Neighbors, local businesspeople, and other
people in your community can also become part of
your support network.

*Joseph used to hang out in Mr. Leone's restaurant
after school every day. There wasn't much else to do,
and he'd rather stay away from home than risk
another beating from his dad.*

*Joseph never said much. He just ordered his usual
soda and sat at one of the back tables until closing
time. One quiet afternoon, he walked to the counter
that Mr. Leone was wiping with his rag. Today had
been a rough day, and Joseph was in a sad mood.
Mr. Leone looked up from the counter and said,
"Young man, can I help you?"*

*Joseph's heart was pounding. He really needed to
tell someone about his problems. But could he talk to
this stranger?*

*Something in Mr. Leone's eyes told Joseph he could
trust the restaurant owner. Soon Joseph found
himself telling Mr. Leone about his dad's drinking
problem and the mess at home.*

*Mr. Leone listened to the whole story. He told
Joseph about his own dad. Then Mr. Leone gave
Joseph the telephone number for Alateen, a group for*

*teenagers whose parents abuse alcohol. Mr. Leone
also offered Joseph a job in the restaurant to help
him save money for college.*

Because he was willing to approach an adult he
trusted, Joseph was able to create one more link in
his support system.

It isn't always easy to take a chance. Asking
other people for help can be scary. But you can
get the support you need if you make an effort to
reach out.

You don't have to pour out your life troubles to
everyone you meet. But think about people in your
community whom you admire and trust. Perhaps
your next-door neighbor seems like a good
listener. Have you always respected the woman
who owns the laundromat down the street? If you
want their support, ask if they'll be willing to talk
with you about your problems.

Very often you'll get a positive response. Many
people want to help you. Sometimes they just don't
know you need their support.

Communication Is the Key!

Good communication skills are important for
you to build a strong support system. Some
individuals are lucky to have people around who
offer help and guidance without being asked.
But for most people, creating a support system

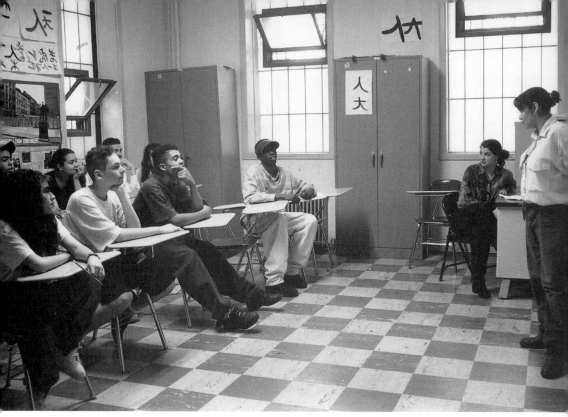

Speaking in front of groups is an excellent way to practice communication skills.

takes work. One of the most important tools you need is the ability to communicate effectively.

Other people can't usually read your mind. In order to help you, they need to know what kind of support you want and when you want it. Sometimes it's hard to ask for help. If you're afraid that other people will laugh at you or ignore you, you may not want to say anything. But the only way you can let them know you need help is by talking to them.

It might be easiest for you to start by asking people you trust. If you feel lonely because your house is empty after school, tell your mom that

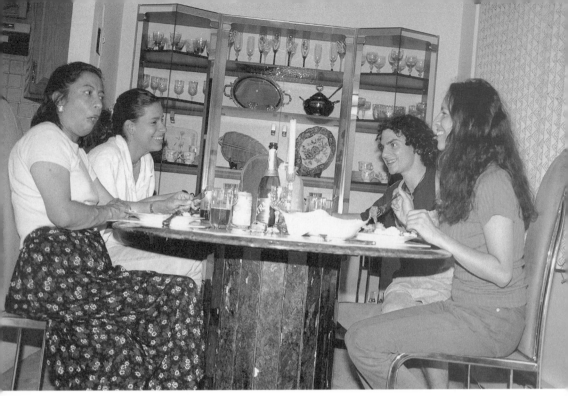

The first place you look to for support may be your own family.

you would like to spend some time alone with her in the evening after she gets home from work.

You can use the same approach with people outside your family. The best way to get support is to be very direct and open.

Explain what you want and how you think the other person can help you. Treat the people you ask with respect—even if they don't always give you what you need.

Tom wanted to earn extra money and learn how to set up his own business. Tom admired his best friend's father, Mr. Ramirez, who had run his own carpentry business for ten years.

Tom decided to telephone Mr. Ramirez. He explained that he was a good student in shop class and someday wanted to become a carpenter. Tom told Mr. Ramirez that he would like to find work now as a carpenter's assistant.

Mr. Ramirez listened carefully to Tom's story. He explained to Tom how he started his own company and helped it grow into a large business. Mr. Ramirez said that he wasn't hiring any workers now, but he offered to introduce Tom to the president of a construction company who needed part-time employees.

Tom got what he wanted because he was willing to ask for help. Even though Mr. Ramirez couldn't offer Tom a job, he was able to introduce Tom to someone else who could.

If you have a strong support system that includes a variety of people, at least one person will probably be able to give you what you want.

You will not always get help or guidance. Hearing "no" can be painful. But if you make wise choices in the people you approach, you will usually end up hearing "yes" more often. And remember that you'll never hear yes if you don't ask.

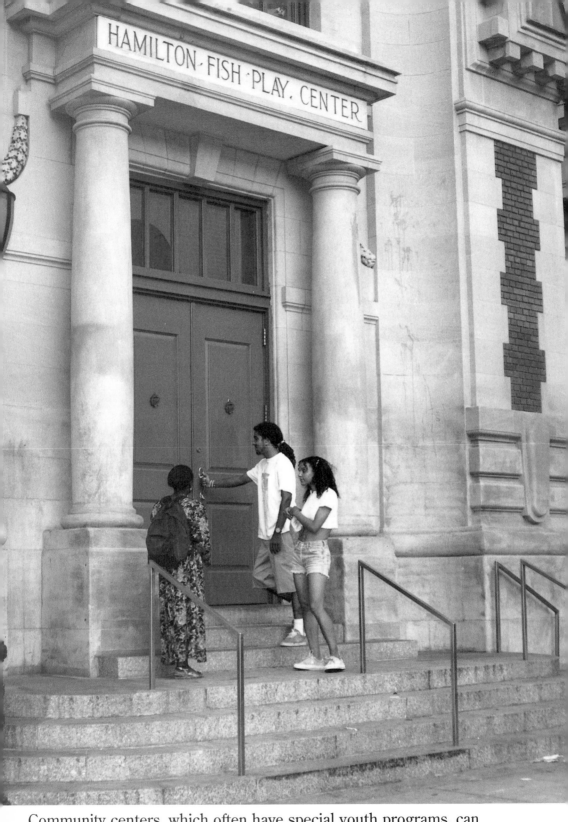

Community centers, which often have special youth programs, can
be good places to meet new people.

Chapter 5

Finding New People

With more than five billion people on the globe, it seems hard to imagine how anyone could feel alone.

But it isn't always easy to meet people and create a strong support system.

One of the keys to developing a strong support system is to get involved with others on a regular schedule. It's hard to form lasting connections with people you meet only occasionally.

Once you have established strong ties with another person, you don't necessarily have to see him or her often for that person to remain a part of your support system. Suppose you and your brother have always been close. If he moves across the country to go to college, you can still turn to him for advice. A good relationship can last for years and years. As long as you still feel you can trust and support each other, you can stay part of each other's support system forever.

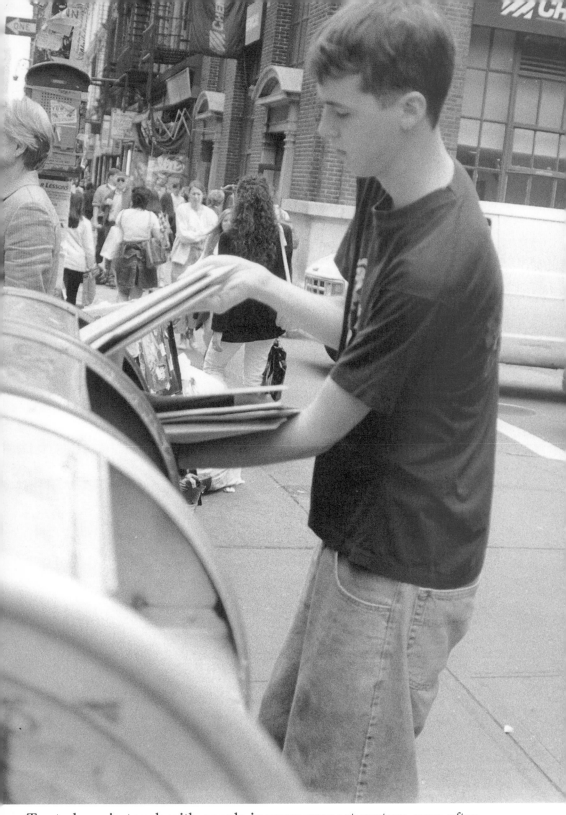

Try to keep in touch with people in your support system even after they have given you the help you need.

In the beginning you need to get to know the people who will become part of your support system. It takes time to develop trust and establish a strong relationship.

You can start building your network by relying on people you know and see regularly. A good place to begin is your school. You go there five days a week and have known many of your classmates and teachers for years. So you probably have a good idea already about which of them you want to include in your support system.

Has Joe always seemed like a person you could trust? Ask him to have lunch with you next Wednesday or invite him to your house after school.

Teachers and guidance counselors are other people in school who can help you. You can build on your existing relationships with them to develop a stronger support system. Set aside a time to talk to them about your educational goals or family problems. They're there to help you.

If you want to build your network, it's important to be consistent. You can get to know people by volunteering once a week at the local hospital, attending regular meetings at the youth center, or getting a part-time job three days a week after school. When you see people regularly, you are more likely to establish strong relationships with them.

You may find that you want to add to your support system. How can you meet new people?

Until last month Hilton was a frustrated and lonely musician. He loved music. He spent hours playing the drums at home. But nobody ever listened to him.

One day Hilton noticed an advertisement on a bulletin board at school. It said the school band was looking for new players. Hilton figured he would try out.

The band leader invited Hilton to join the band. Hilton loves going to band twice a week and performing at local parties and fairs. Other people enjoy the music Hilton makes. And they like Hilton too. He's become friends with other members of the band.

Classes, Clubs, and Community Centers

You can build your support system by joining groups of people who have interests similar to yours. You might get involved with a theater group or take an art class.

Think about your skills and talents. Do you enjoy sports? You might join one of your school's athletic teams. You don't have to be a professional athlete: You could play on an intramural team or look for a regular volleyball game at the local YMCA or community center.

"But I don't have any special skills," you say to yourself. That's not true. Everyone has talents.

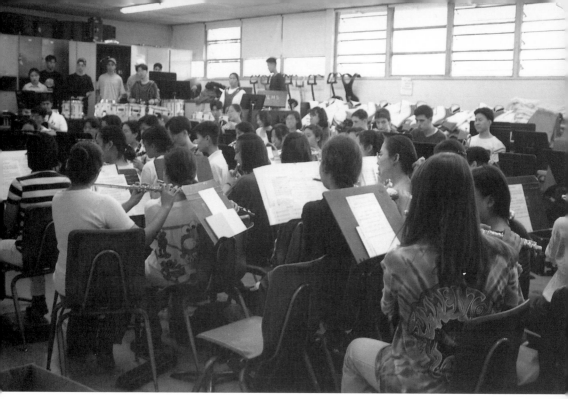

Improve on an existing skill or start a new hobby by joining a school activity.

Would you like to develop your abilities? You might take an art class at a youth center or learn how to fix bicycles.

By getting involved in a group, you'll meet other people with similar interests. You'll be able to talk to them about the things you have in common. Learning a new skill will also increase your self-esteem. You can be proud of yourself for mastering a new task.

Your school, community center, or 4-H club might also have programs to help you prepare for your career. Perhaps you'll join a group like Future Farmers of America. Some local businesses create partnerships with schools to help students

47

who want to become entrepreneurs and own their own companies someday.

Would you like a medical career? Many hospitals have volunteer opportunities or groups for students who want to learn about careers in health care.

If you don't have a particular career choice or special interest, you might join a group with a more general focus to meet people your own age.

Your local YMCA, community center, Scouts, or Boys and Girls Clubs sponsor many activities, classes, and social events where you can meet other people. You'll gain confidence and make friends by interacting with other people and talking about yourself and your interests.

"I was new to the neighborhood and didn't know where to meet people," said Jeff. "All of the kids at school seemed to know everyone else already. I couldn't join the band because I don't play an instrument, and I don't really have any hobbies.

"Finally I decided to check out the after-school program at the youth center here. I'm glad I did. Now I've gotten to know a bunch of other kids.

"Sometimes we just hang out. But we also talk about our problems. And a few of us are thinking of starting our own T-shirt business to make some extra money.

"I feel better about myself since I started coming here. And now I'm not as lonely."

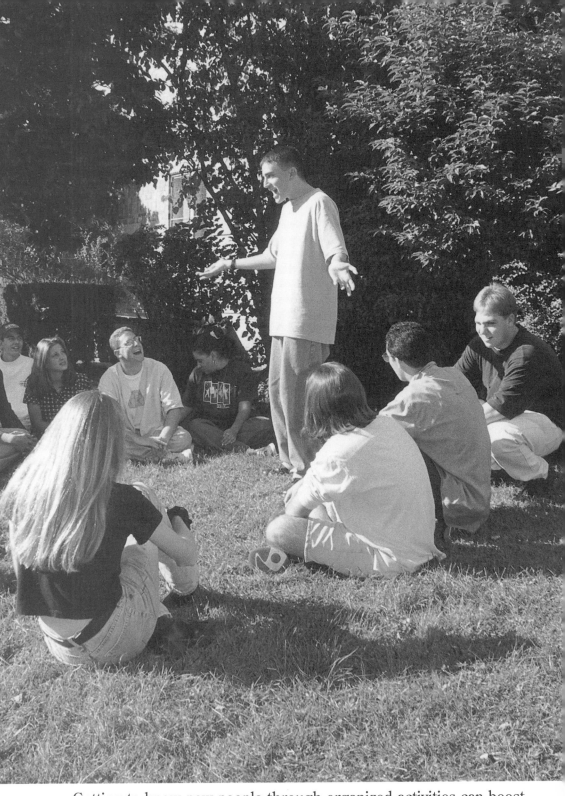

Getting to know new people through organized activities can boost your self-esteem and make you more comfortable communicating with others.

Helping Groups

Sometimes teens without a support system turn to drugs or alcohol. Using these substances can often make your problems worse.

But there are people who can help you. Alcoholics Anonymous, Narcotics Anonymous, and other programs are designed to provide support for people who abuse alcohol and other drugs. Joining one of these groups can help you with both of your problems: overcoming your dependence on drugs or alcohol and building a strong support system.

Your school or community center may also run programs for people with these problems.

"I thought I was the only person who drank when I got lonely. After talking with other people in my group, I know that a lot of other people feel the same way. Now I'm learning other methods to handle my problems," said one teenage member of Alcoholics Anonymous.

Many people find that becoming part of a group of people with the same problem helps them feel better. The members of these groups have experienced many of the same situations. They can help one another get through the rough times together.

In addition to groups for substance abusers, there are also support groups for people with many other problems. Survivors of incest, rape, or

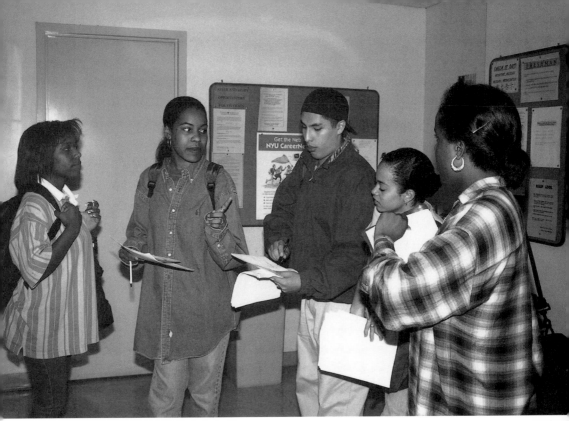

Seek out information at school about support groups that may be available for students with specific problems.

domestic abuse and people with eating disorders often join self-help or therapy groups.

Sometimes people with other physical or mental problems join together too. Hospitals or medical centers often have classes or meetings for people with diabetes or mental disorders. The patients and their families talk about their problems. Members also discuss positive experiences and successful methods they have used to cope with new challenges.

Many people find that these groups help them build a strong support network. But you may not

feel comfortable talking about your problems in
front of many people. You can still use your
support network. Talk to a counselor at school or
a local health center. They can provide
encouragement and help you deal with your drug
and alcohol abuse. When you are having a hard
time, knowing someone else cares about you can
help you go a long way toward overcoming your
problems.

Finding a Mentor

Some of the people in your support system will
be your own age. It's good to have friends you can
talk to about your problems and with whom you
can share your experiences.

But older people may also be an important part
of your support network. Often they can use their
experiences and knowledge to help you set goals
and solve problems.

Some communities have mentoring programs
like Big Brothers/Big Sisters. A youth leader in
your community center might also be a mentor for
you.

*"I really like having Michelle as my Big Sister,"
said one teen. "She's only a few years older than I
am, so she knows what I'm going through. I can talk
to her about boyfriends, school problems, or just
about anything. She's terrific."*

You don't have to be part of a formal program to have a mentor. Often local businesspeople or neighbors are very happy to help you.

"I'd always admired Mr. Garcetti," said Jason. "He owns his own clothing store, has a family, and seems to lead a pretty good life. Someday I want to start my own company. But I had no idea where to start.

"I finally decided to talk to him. I was nervous, but he was so nice. He answered all of my questions. Now I go to talk to him at least once a week. He's become almost like a second father to me."

How can you find a mentor? First you might look for announcements in the newspaper or on television or radio about Big Brother/Big Sister programs. Sometimes these programs may be advertised at the library or youth center in your community.

Ask your guidance counselor or teachers if they know about any programs. You might also ask at your church or synagogue. Check the yellow pages of your telephone book under "Youth Organizations."

If your school doesn't have a mentoring program in place, you might want to talk to your principal, guidance counselor, or favorite teacher about starting a project. Once the staff members know that students are interested, they may be very eager to work with you to get one started.

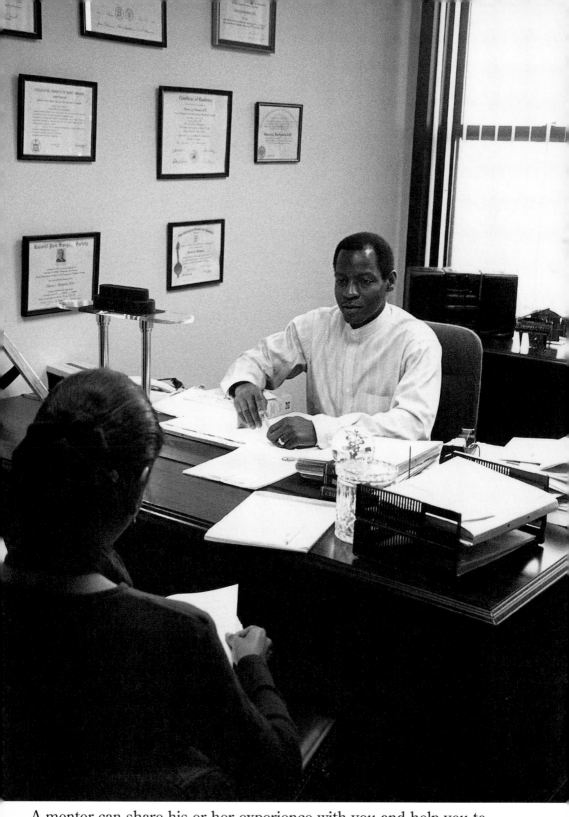

A mentor can share his or her experience with you and help you to gain insight on a certain job or profession.

But you don't need to join a program to find an adult mentor. First, decide what you want to learn from this person. Do you need help in developing your job skills? Are you looking for someone in whom you can confide?

Think about the adults you know and admire. If you have a particular job in mind, consider people you know who work in that field. If you want your mentor to serve as a more general advisor, make a list of the people in your community whom you trust and admire.

Once you have decided who would make a good mentor for you, set up a time to talk to the person. Explain why you want a mentor. Be respectful and direct so that the person understands what you want and how he or she could help you.

The person may be very glad to take on the role. You and your mentor may decide to schedule regular meeting times, or the two of you might prefer a more informal arrangement.

Sometimes the people you ask for help may say no. They may not have the time to make a regular commitment. But even if they don't become your "official" mentors, they will probably still be willing to talk to you when they have time. And they may be able to suggest other people who would be willing to become mentors for you.

A good mentor can be an important part of your support system. Your mentor will teach you new skills and provide emotional support.

Your mentor can offer guidance, make
suggestions about ways you might improve or
build on your talents, and help you establish and
reach your goals.

*Because her mother works long hours, Dana used
to spend hours alone every day after school. Finally
Dana decided to ask her next-door neighbor, who
makes and sells jewelry from her home, if she would
serve as Dana's adviser.*

*"Mrs. Josephson is an excellent mentor," said
Dana. "She's teaching me how to make bracelets
and necklaces, and she's always willing to offer
suggestions when I tell her my problems. I'd like to
open my own store someday, and I'm learning the
skills I'll need by watching how she operates her
business."*

A mentor can be a very valuable part of your
support system. But you will also help your
mentor by becoming part of his or her support
system. "I love having Dana around," said Mrs.
Josephson. "She's quick to learn, and she's been a
big help to me in running the business. Even more
important, she has a wonderful personality, and I
enjoy spending time with her."

Many teens establish strong ties with their
mentors. And the relationship can often give you a
big push forward in meeting your goals.

In 1981, New York businessman Eugene Lang

became the mentor for 61 sixth-graders in the graduating class of PS 121, the elementary school he had attended as a boy. PS 121 had a high drop-out rate. But five years after Mr. Lang became their mentor, almost all of the students were still in school. Nearly half of the students went on to college. And many of the others found good jobs, thanks to the advice and support of Mr. Lang.

He's a good example of a supportive mentor!

If you've had a good relationship with an advisor, you may decide to return the favor and become a mentor for a younger student. Both of you will benefit. Your "mentee" will gain confidence and new skills from you, and you'll feel good about yourself since you know you'll be helping someone who needs your support.

Returning the Favor

Rememember Charlie in the Introduction? After that sad morning Charlie knew it was time to make some changes. He went to the local community center to see what he could do with his time. At first he decided just to play basketball after school.

Soon he became a regular player on an intramural team. Then he signed up for a woodworking class.

When he saw an announcement for a mentoring program, Charlie put his name on the list. The program matched him with a neighborhood carpenter who owns his own business. Every week Charlie spends time with the carpenter, who helps Charlie develop his skills and listens when Charlie needs to talk about his problems at home.

Charlie feels better about his life today. He plans to go to vocational school after he gets his high-school diploma and maybe open his own shop someday. His home life is still rocky, but he's glad he can depend on someone else to help him through the rough spots.

Charlie will graduate from high school next week. He's excited about continuing his education. And he's made a special commitment. He's going to become a Big Brother for a junior high school student.

"It's not easy to make it out there on your own," he said recently. *"Other people have helped me get where I am today. Now it's my turn to help someone else."*

"There are so many people who care. No one should have to feel alone."

Help List

The organizations listed here are national groups. They may be able to provide information about local branches in your community. Also, look in the white pages of your telephone book for local groups and check the yellow pages under "Youth Groups" or "Youth Organizations."

Big Brothers/Big Sisters of America
230 North 13th Street
Philadelphia, PA 19107
(215) 567-1000
e–mail: bbbsa@aol.com

Boys and Girls Clubs of America
771 First Avenue
New York, NY 10017
(404) 815-5700

Junior Achievement Inc.
1 Education Way
Colorado Springs, CO 80906
(719) 636-2474

National Association for Industry-Education
    Cooperation
235 Hendricks Boulevard
Buffalo, NY 14266
(716) 834-7047

United Way of America
701 North Fairfax Street
Alexandria, VA 22314–2045
(703) 836-7100

For information about Alcoholics Anonymous, Narcotics Anonymous, Al-Anon and other support groups, look for a local listing in your telephone book.

Boy Scouts of America
1325 West Walnut Hill Lane
PO Box 152079
Irving, TX 75015-2079
(214) 580-2000
Internet: http://www.bsa.scouting.org

NAACP Youth and College Division
4805 Mount Hope Drive
Baltimore, MD 21215—3297
(410) 448-3722

Vocational Industrial Clubs of America
PO Box 3000
Leesburg, VA 22075
(703) 777-8810
e–mail: dialogvica@aol.com

In Canada:

Big Brothers and Sisters of Canada
5230 South Service Road
Burlington, Ontario L7L 5K2
(905) 639-0461
e–mail: bbsc@bbsc.ca

Girl Guides of Canada
50 Merton Street
Toronto, ON M4S IAS
(800) 565-5281

Scouts Canada
National Council
1345 Baseline Road
Ottawa, ON K2C 3G7
(613) 224-5134
e–mail: scouts.ca

Glossary—*Explaining New Words*

emotional support   Guidance, encouragement, sympathy, and advice.

entrepreneur   A person who starts his or her own business.

goal   Something you want to accomplish; an aim; an objective.

mentor   An advisor or older person who offers guidance and support.

network   An interlocking system; a network of people and groups who help you.

role models   People whom you admire and whose behavior you try to copy.

self-esteem   The feelings you have about yourself and your value.

strategy   Plan for accomplishing a goal.

support system   People or groups in your life who provide emotional help, guidance, and education.

vocational guidance   Information and advice about your career and job plans.

For Further Reading

American Association of Higher Education. *National Directory of School-College Partnerships: Current Models and Practices.* 1987.

One-to-One Partnership, Inc. *Guide to Workplace Mentoring Programs.* Washington, DC: 1992.

McFarland, Rhoda. *The World of Work.* New York: The Rosen Publishing Group, 1993.

Milios, Rita. *Independent Living.* New York: The Rosen Publishing Group, 1992.

Rigden, Diana W. *Business and the Schools: A Guide to Effective Programs.* New York: Council for Aid to Education, 1992.

Smith, Sandra Lee. *Setting Goals.* New York: The Rosen Publishing Group, 1992.

Index

About the Author
Anna Kreiner is the author of *Everything You Need to Know About School Violence*, *In Control: Saying No to Sexual Pressure*, *Let's Talk About Being Afraid*, and *Let's Talk About Drug Abuse*.

Photo Credits
Cover photo by Michael Brandt.
Photographs on page 49, 54: Katherine Hsu. All other photos: Maria Moreno.